HOMOEOPATHY
and
IMMUNIZATION

compiled by
LESLIE J. SPEIGHT

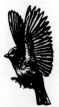

THE C. W. DANIEL COMPANY LTD
1 CHURCH PATH, SAFFRON WALDEN,
ESSEX CB10 1JP, ENGLAND

First Edition 1982
Second Edition 1983
Reprinted 1985
Third Edition 1987
Reprinted 1995

The Random House Group Limited supports The Forest Stewardship
Council (FSC®), the leading international forest certification organisation.
Our books carrying the FSC label are printed on FSC® certified paper.
FSC is the only forest certification scheme endorsed by the leading
environmental organisations, including Greenpeace. Our
paper procurement policy can be found at
www.randomhouse.co.uk/environment

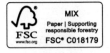

MIX
Paper | Supporting
responsible forestry
FSC
www.fsc.org   FSC® C018179

Printed and bound in Great Britain by Clays Ltd, St Ives PLC

ISBN 0 85032 199 9

Set by MS Typesetting, Castle Camps, Cambridge

INTRODUCTION

The increasing public awareness of the dangers associated with some immunizations is arousing great apprehension in many parents. They are questioning the long term effects in spite of the widely recommended procedures by health authorities and doctors.

Many years ago Dr. J. Compton Burnett, a famous homoeopathic doctor, wrote a book entitled 'Vaccinosis' in which he pointed out the ill effects and dangers of vaccination. Since that time immunizations have become commonplace on the assumption that they can prevent the development of a disease. It must be borne in mind, however, that there is no proof that any individual will develop it in the first place.

Statistics are often produced purporting to show that the incidence of a disease has decreased after the introduction of immunization, but diseases have a habit of running in cycles and there is always the possibility of a decrease coinciding with the use of the alleged immunizing agent.

The body has a built-in immunity system and if this is strengthened by good food and satisfactory living conditions, it can play an important role in resisting any epidemic and, in fact, any disease which might attack those who ignore these important factors.

Occasionally there is a report of irreparable damage caused by immunization. Minor effects are not publicised even if they are recognised as being the result of the inoculation which introduces foreign matter into the body.

In homoeopathy there is no immunization as such, but there are remedies that can build up immunity to infections. They can also act as curative agents where a disease has developed. These remedies carry no risk of detrimental effects, they are absolutely safe.

Dr. A. Pulford wrote 'No disease will arise without an existing predisposition to that disease. It is the absence of the predisposition to any particular disease that makes us immune to it. Homoeopathy alone is capable of removing these predispositions. '

The homoeopathic prophylaxis will immunize for 3 to 4 weeks so it should be repeated at the outbreak of another epidemic.

Dr. Dorothy Shepherd states that a homoeopathic preparation of the whooping cough bacillus was administered daily for two weeks to 364 cases after contact with the disease and not one child developed whooping cough. Another homoeopathic physician gave Lathyrus Sativa to 82 people who were in close proximity to the suspect area of poliomyelitis with 12 people being direct contacts. There were 63 children and 19 adults in the group and not one developed the disease.

CHICKEN POX

Early symptoms are an eruption on the trunk, chest and back spreading to the arms and face, usually thicker on the shoulders and upper arms than on wrists and hands. More on thighs than on legs and feet.

Fresh crops of spots appear every two days before or simultaneously with a rise in temperature. There are clear blisters on the skin together with dried up crusts and scabs.

Homoeopathic Prophylaxis

VARICELLA 30, one pill or tablet at 4 hourly intervals for 3 doses in one day. Then one dose weekly while there is a risk of infection.

CHOLERA

This is a disease in which homoeopathy has achieved great success. The death rate under orthodox treatment is very high and statistics giving comparisons of the mortality under the two systems emphasize the superiority of homoeopathic treatment. The early symptoms are usually painless diarrhoea accompanied by sudden prostration and sudden coldness.

Homoeopathic Prophylaxis

RUBINI'S CAMPHOR, 2 or 3 drops on a piece of sugar once or twice a day (it can cause nausea if taken in water).

In addition one or two drops of CUPRUM ACETICUM 3x in a little water may be given night and morning where a person is much exposed to the disease.

Under the heading 'Prevention' Dr. John H. Clarke in his 'Prescriber' says "Wear near the skin a plate of copper (6 in. by 4, for a man of large size; 5 in. by 3 for a small man, and for a woman; 4 in. by 2 for children). Let it be fastened round the waist by straps attached to longitudinal slits cut in the ends of the plate, which should be oval. Let the plate rest in front of the abdominal wall and let it be made slightly concave, so as to adapt itself to the shape of the body. The plate should be worn day and night. It may be cleaned from time to time by rubbing with vinegar."

Where this disease is prevalent hygiene is most important. Rooms should be dry, clean and well aired. Exposure to cold and wet should be avoided.

As homoeopathic treatment is so successful in dealing with this very serious ailment it is always wise to consult a homoeopathic doctor if cholera is suspected.

Dr. Shepherd mentions three 'classic' remedies – Camphor, Cuprum and Veratrum alb., which have proved invaluable when prescribed according to the symptoms. There are, however, other remedies that must be considered when treating this disease.

DIPHTHERIA

Commences with a sore throat and the tonsils and larynx become involved. The membrane of the throat has a glistening gelatinous appearance, the breath has a sickening smell, there is headache and a general feeling of malaise.

Any suspicion of paralysis should be reported to a doctor immediately.

One source of information states that the vaccine seems to be very effective but that, in very rare instances, may cause polio. Another says there is some doubt about its efficacy.

Homoeopathic Prophylaxis

DIPHTHERINUM 30, one pill or tablet at 4 hourly intervals for 3 doses in one day. Then one dose weekly while there is a risk of infection.

Dr. Grimmer, a famous homoeopathic physician, recommended PYROGEN. If the first mentioned remedy is not available immediately take this in the same dosage.

GERMAN MEASLES

Children with this disease display mild symptoms of fever, rash and tiredness. The risk of serious complications is rare.

A significant proportion of mothers who had this complaint during the first three months of pregnancy often produced babies with deformities, eye defects, deafness and mental retardation.

In addition to the protection of children, women of child-bearing age are often given the vaccine if they haven't adequate antibodies in their blood. The vaccine can cause a rash, swollen lymph nodes and pains in the joints, usually between 2 and 10 weeks after the immunization.

Homoeopathic Prophylaxis

RUBELLA 30, one pill or tablet at 4 hourly intervals for 3 doses in one day. Subsequently one dose weekly if there is still risk of infection.

If Rubella is not available immediately take PULSATILLA 12 or 30 in the same dosage.

INFLUENZA

When there is an epidemic of this common trouble take one pill or tablet of INFLUENZINUM 30 night and morning for 3 days. Repeat at weekly intervals while there is a risk.

Some homoeopathic chemists offer two homoeopathic remedies in combination – *Influenzinum* and *Bacillinum* – which seems to be effective. They would advise regarding dosage.

MEASLES

A highly contagious disease characterised by cold symptoms, cough, irritation of the eyes and high fever. A rash appears on the fourth day of the illness. There can be complications such as ear infections, pneumonia and infection of the lymph nodes.

There has been an impressive decline in this complaint since the introduction of the vaccine but there is statistical evidence showing that many cases occur after the vaccination. Some children develop a fever and there are reports of severe reactions of the central nervous system in a few instances.

Martin Weitz in 'Health Shock' states 'Strong reactions of the vaccine are not uncommon. In one survey 32 per cent of children had a general reaction (such as fever and skin rash), which was severe in 6 per cent. But the risk of neurological disorders, i.e. brain damage, is very low according to an American survey of 51 million children vaccinated. It occurred about once in every 600,000 cases. It should not be given to children sensitive to egg protein or those with a history of convulsions, TB or cancer.'

Homoeopathic Prophylaxis

MORBILLINUM 30, one pill or tablet at 4 hourly intervals for 3 doses in one day. Then one dose weekly until the trouble has passed.

If only the 12th potency is available give in the same dosage. In the 200th potency this remedy should be taken once a week for 3 doses.

If the above mentioned is not at hand PULSATILLA 12 or 30 should be given as prescribed for *Morbillinum* 12 and 30.

In many cases *Morbillinum* will help to clear any after effects of measles.

MUMPS

A highly contagious disease commencing with a fever associated with the parotid gland. In addition there is headache and tiredness. Within 24 hours there is earache near the lobe of the ear and the next day the salivary glands in front of the ear become swollen. Pain during mastication and on opening of the mouth. The illness runs its course within 6 days.

In adults there can be orchitis, inflammation of the testicles, ovaries etc. These troubles occur much less frequently in children.

The vaccine seems to give immunity in a very high percentage of cases.

Homoeopathic Prophylaxis

PAROTIDINUM 30 one pill or tablet at 4 hourly intervals for 3 doses in one day.

For the after effects of mumps *Pilocarpine* 6 night and morning should be given for a few days but stopped as soon as an improvement commences and not repeated unless the symptoms recur.

POLIO

The incidence of this much feared disease has decreased dramatically and the vaccine has, apparently, brought about this decline. However, it seems that there are risks; pregnant women should not be vaccinated as it causes a 20% increase in the risk of stillbirths during the first four months of pregnancy.

Polio should always be under the care of a doctor (homoeopathic if possible).

Dr. Grimmer recommends *Lathyrus Sativus* 30 or 200 once every three weeks during an epidemic and he claims that there will be no case of paralysis.

Another homoeopathic remedy that seems to cover the symptoms of polio is *Gelsemium.*

SCARLET FEVER

There are very few cases but the onset of this very contagious disease is abrupt, commencing with vomiting, fever and sore throat. The mucous membrane of the throat is bright red, the tongue is furred with enlarged inflamed papillae showing through the white edges. A skin rash appears within 24 hours with bright red face and it spreads all over the body.

If neglected there can be serious complications but homoeopathy has several most effective remedies and it is advisable to consult a homoeopathic physician as soon as the trouble is suspected.

Homoeopathic Prophylaxis

SCARLATINUM 30, one pill or tablet at 4 hourly intervals for 3 doses in one day. Then one dose at weekly intervals for 3 weeks.

SMALL-POX

The first symptoms are severe backache, intense headache and fever. Also a dirty tongue and deranged stomach. At the commencement the eruption is similar to that of measles but if the finger is passed over the skin there is a feeling – as if fine shot were under the skin.

Homoeopathic Prophylaxis

VARIOLINUM 6 or 30, one pill or tablet night and morning during the trouble. An alternative remedy is MALANDRINUM 30 in the same dosage.

TYPHOID

Caused mainly by lack of cleanliness and bad sanitation. The utmost care should be exercised when handling food – the hands should be scrupulously clean and all food in shops and in the home should be covered to prevent flies contaminating it. Lavatories used by sufferers should be thoroughly disinfected and in places where water is suspect it is advisable to drink only the bottled variety.

Homoeopathic Prophylaxis

TYPHOIDINUM 30, one pill or tablet at 4 hourly intervals for three doses in a day. This may be continued throughout the epidemic.

TYPHUS

Another dirt disease which is usually controlled by cleanliness. Can be passed from one sufferer to another by carrier lice.

Cleanliness is of paramount importance; infected rooms should be disinfected and re-papered.

Homoeopathic Prophylaxis

All the authorities consulted stress the importance of cleanliness and omit to mention remedies. However, one reliable source recommends HYOSCYAMUS or BAPTISIA. One pill or tablet of either in the 12th potency, night and morning, should be taken for several days.

Repeat if considered advisable.

WHOOPING COUGH

An infectious disease of childhood which can sometimes have alarming symptoms. Usually the child appears to have a cold followed by violent coughing for four to six weeks. This mainly occurs in infants and young children.

Deaths are usually due to complicating respiratory troubles. Pneumonia is responsible for a very high proportion of deaths in children under three years of age.

There was a great reduction in the mortality from this disease before the vaccine was introduced. There is conflicting evidence regarding the results of immunization, one report mentions that of 85 fully immunized children at least 46 developed whooping cough.

Homoeopathic Prophylaxis

Immediately there is any risk of contact give one pill or tablet of PERTUSSIN 30 night and morning once a week for 6 to 8 weeks.

PLEASE READ THESE NOTES

When it is impossible to administer a pill or tablet dissolve one pill or crushed tablet in a small wineglass of cold water and give a teaspoonful as a dose.

It is unnecessary to give more than one pill or tablet as a dose although more will do no harm.

Do not repeat the suggested dose unless absolutely necessary as the medicines can work in the body for a considerable time and too frequent repetition can interfere with the curative action.

Homoeopathic medicines are produced by potentisation which renders them sensitive to strong sunlight, odours etc. They should be stored in a cool, dark place away from strong perfumes, scented soap, lipstick, peppermint etc.

When taking the medicines refrain from coffee and strong drinks such as peppermint tea.

Pills and tablets should be allowed to dissolve under the tongue and not be washed down with liquid.

Combinations of homoeopathic medicines are often offered as specifics for a variety of ailments but they cannot be truly homoeopathic as the basic principle of homoeopathy is to individualize. The remedy that has produced similar symptoms in a healthy person must be given. The name of the disease is not important in this scientific method of treatment, except for convenience in describing the patient's condition. When a combination of remedies is given without success homoeopathy is often condemned as useless, a totally unfair assessment.

This small booklet deals only with remedies that act as prophylactics but, at all times, it is advisable to consult a competent homoeopath as soon as trouble is suspected. Homoeopathy can not only act as a preventative but as a most efficient curative method in all ailments, even those deep-seated troubles often considered incurable by other means.

Remember that medicine cannot eradicate symptoms caused by unwise actions such as smoking, poor food, lack of exercise, excessive drinking of alcohol, lack of fresh air etc.

The preparation of homoeopathic medicines is a job for the specialist and, in consequence, it is advisable, at all times, to obtain remedies from a reputable homoeopathic pharmacy.

Most homoeopathic pharmacies supply cases containing ten or twelve bottles of any selected remedies. I have just received one from Ainsworth's Homoeopathic Pharmacy, 38 New Cavendish Street, London, W1M 7LH containing Varicella 30, Diphtherinum 30, Rubella 30, Influenzinum 30, Morbillinum 30, Parotidinum 30, Scarlatinum 30, Pertussin 30, Arnica 30 and Nux Vomica 30.

Arnica should be in every home and given in any accident (it not only deals with bruising but removes the shock, which is so important), overtiredness from excessive exertion, sprains, after tooth extraction and operations.

Nux Vomica gives great relief to people who over-eat and over indulge in alcohol—it clears up 'morning after the night before' feeling very quickly. It has many uses which are given in any materia medica.

When ordering a case of medicines the remedies and potencies should be named.

I hope this small work will be of help to many and save much suffering.

Leslie J. Speight

P.S. There is no standard dosage in homoeopathy. Those who wish to take additional precautions could supplement the suggested dosage by taking one pill or tablet of the same remedy on three consecutive days and repeat this at 3, 6, 9 or 12 monthly intervals.

THE FOLLOWING BOOKS ARE RECOMMENDED FOR THOSE WISHING FOR MORE KNOWLEDGE ABOUT HOMOEOPATHY

HOMOEOPATHY IN EPIDEMIC DISEASES by Dr. Dorothy Shepherd. Enables those far from homoeopathic help to deal with epidemic diseases.

HOMOEOPATHY, A GUIDE TO NATURAL MEDICINE by Phyllis Speight. Excellent for those with no knowledge of the subject.

PUDDEPHATT'S PRIMERS by Noel Puddephatt, revised and re-arranged by Phyllis Speight. Originally three small booklets entitled 'First Steps to Homoeopathy', 'How To Find The Correct Remedy' and 'The Homoeopathic Materia Medica, How It Should be Studied'.

ARNICA THE WONDER HERB by Phyllis Speight. Probably the best ambassador for homoeopathy, giving details of the most commonly used remedy in a great number of everyday troubles.

A STUDY COURSE IN HOMOEOPATHY by Phyllis Speight and THE PRINCIPLES & ART OF CURE BY HOMOEOPATHY by Dr. H. A. Roberts. These two works studied together give a deep understanding of the basis of homoeopathy.

All of the above are available from The C. W. Daniel Company Ltd.

PERTINENT QUESTIONS

and

ANSWERS

about

HOMOEOPATHY

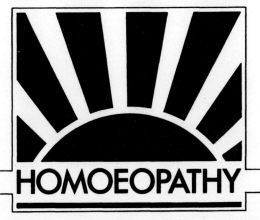

PERTINENT QUESTIONS

and

ANSWERS

about

HOMOEOPATHY

Phyllis Speight

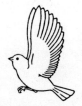

Health Science Press
The C. W. Daniel Company Ltd
1 Church Path, Saffron Walden, Essex, England

By the same Author

Arnica the Wonder Herb
Before Calling the Doctor
A Comparison of the Chronic Miasms
Homoeopathy, A Practical Guide to Natural Medicine
Homoeopathy for Emergencies
Homoeopathic Remedies for Children
Overcoming Rheumatism and Arthritis
A Study Course in Homoeopathy
Homoeopathic Remedies for Womens' Ailments

© *Phyllis Speight*
1984
Reprinted January 1987
ISBN 085207 164 7

Cover design by Craige Quainton
Typeset in Souvenir Medium and Bold

The Random House Group Limited supports The Forest Stewardship
Council (FSC®), the leading international forest certification organisation.
Our books carrying the FSC label are printed on FSC® certified paper.
FSC is the only forest certification scheme endorsed by the leading
environmental organisations, including Greenpeace. Our
paper procurement policy can be found at
www.randomhouse.co.uk/environment

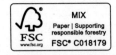

MIX
Paper | Supporting
responsible forestry
FSC
www.fsc.org   FSC® C018179

Printed and bound in Great Britain by Clays Ltd, St Ives PLC

CONTENTS

INTRODUCTION

At the end of any lecture on homoeopathy there are numerous questions which often prove of great interest and help to those seeking an understanding of the subject.

The questions and answers given here are a selection of the most important from a series of lectures given by my wife.

Information in this form is easy to absorb and it should prove of value to those who are unable, or unwilling, to make a study of the text books which give information in great detail but do not provide all the answers!

Leslie J. Speight

1. Why is Homoeopathy preferable to orthodox (Allopathic) treatment?

Because it aims to cure the patient by eradicating the cause of the trouble.

When correctly prescribed the remedies never suppress symptoms.

Homoeopathic remedies **never** cause side effects. Once a remedy is fully proven it is used for all time to cure symptoms brought out in the provings. Our remedies are taken orally and there is no unpleasant taste, a great advantage when prescribing for children.

2. With which diseases can Homoeopathy deal?

Dr Clarke once said *Homoeopathy the most complete and scientific system of medicine the world has ever seen.* It is indeed a complete system of medicine and it works in helping the built-in healing mechanism of the patient to do its own curing. Therefore, as the patient becomes better and better, more and more symptoms disappear. This happens whatever the name of the disease.

If a patient is incurable then the same remedies, those that fit the patient, are the best palliatives.

3. Is Homoeopathy effective in mental troubles?

Yes, very, because all symptoms of the mind are so important in an assessment of the remedy. Hahnemann obtained excellent results in mental illness and more recently Dr Dorothy Shepherd wrote about some of her experiences and added that in her opinion 80% of patients in 'Mental Homes' could be cured by homoeopathic medicines. Every homoeopath, I am sure, could give illustrations of patients cured in this field.

4. Can Homoeopathy cure cancer?

I answered this when dealing with the second question.

Cancer is a name given to a certain set of symptoms – this applies to all diseases – and so exactly the same principles are applied.

Homoeopathy has cured many cases of cancer. Unfortunately, the disease is very often not diagnosed until it is in an advanced state and it is then too late for any therapy to cure. Some patients will come for homoeopathic treatment after having tried various therapies and, here again, it is often too late for cure. But I will repeat, homoeopathy can often palliate incurable patients. Never give up hope.

5. Do Homoeopaths approve of surgery?

Sometimes surgery is necessary for drainage purposes and there are times when it saves life but I am of the opinion that surgery is often used when homoeopathy could clear up the condition with medicines.

Many years ago an American surgeon, Dr E. Carleton wrote *Homoeopathy in Medicine & Surgery* in which he gave details of numerous ailments that could usually be dealt with by homoeopathy thus rendering surgery unnecessary.

I would always advise a sufferer to try homoeopathy before agreeing to an operation, however there are times when delay could be dangerous and there is no alternative to surgery.

Throughout the years patients have come to me asking if homoeopathy could help as their doctors had advised an operation, the list covers a wide range from the removal of tonsils and gall-bladders, ruptures, prolapsed conditions, hysterectomies etc., and many were cured without surgery.

When pathological conditions have progressed to the point where medicines are unlikely to be effective surgery may be justified.

6. Can I stop taking drugs whilst having homoeopathic remedies?

This depends upon the drugs. Usually it is dangerous to stop taking drugs suddenly, the withdrawal symptoms are too great. However, after a while on homoeopathic treatment the patient often feels better and then allopathic medicines can gradually be reduced and eventually stopped. It is the aim of every homoeopath to release the patient from drugs.

7. Can homoeopathic remedies do any harm?

Never when used by a homoeopath with knowledge and experience.

When chronic disease is treated there may be an aggravation of symptoms for a short period and this is because our remedies work from the centre to the circumference and so drive out the poisons from the system. **This is the only way to cure**.

Homeopathic remedies **never** cause any side-effects.

8. Can Homoeopathy deal with arthritic deformities?

Very rarely can a deformed joint be returned to normal although pain and swelling can be cleared up.

The deformities are seldom affected although there was a case shown on television (X-Ray) where a deformity of the knee was cured and the joint normal. So never give up hope.

9. How long do homoeopathic remedies work?

It is impossible to give specific times as some work for a much longer period than others. Potencies too must be considered. Low potencies such as 6, 12 and 30 do not work as long as the higher potencies such as the 200th, 1m. etc. A high potency could work for a month or longer, depending upon the patient and the illness.

The golden rule is to cease giving a medicine as soon as an improvement is noticed and only repeat the dose when symp-

11

toms begin to return. In very acute troubles it might be necessary to give a dose every few minutes to bring about a reaction.

10. Which is the best potency to use?

There is no 'best' potency, they all work and in my view all are necessary.

In dealing with chronic disease an experienced homoeopath would endeavour to select the potency most suitable to the patient but in domestic prescribing anyone with little experience should use the 6th, 12th, or 30th potencies. As a general rule the 30th would be required less frequently than the lower ones.

11. Does coffee interfere with the action of homoeopathic remedies?

Much has been written about the antidotal effect of coffee but in my experience I have found that my remedies work as long as they are not taken within half-an-hour of drinking coffee. This does not mean that I approve of anybody drinking endless cups of coffee and if I cannot persuade patients to give it up then I compromise by limiting the consumption to two cups daily.

However there are some homoeopathic remedies that are actually antidoted by coffee and when one of these is prescribed I ask the patient to give up coffee for a period and explain the reason.

12. Do homoeopaths consider Osteopathy helpful?

Yes.

When there is a displacement of bones etc., osteopathy can usually deal with the trouble and the deep massage that some osteopaths apply can be soothing and helfpul.

Where there is soreness after a treatment **Arnica** can help to remove the discomfort.

Osteopaths and homoeopaths work together with excellent results.

13. Are Bach remedies homoeopathic?

No. The preparation of these remedies in no way resembles that of homoeopathic potentisation and the method of arriving at a prescription is entirely different from that of homoeopathy. The belief that these remedies are homoeopathic probably originated from the fact that Dr Bach, at one stage of his career, carried out research at The Royal London Homoeopathic Hospital. Their use is based upon mental symptoms only, whereas homoeopathic treatment takes into account all aspects of the patient.

14. Are herbal remedies related to homoeopathy?

Some homoeopathic remedies are derived from herbal sources but they are not prescribed in the substantial doses used by herbalists, or for the same reasons.

Homoeopathic remedies prepared from herbals start with the mother tincture which is similar to a herbal fluid extract but they are then potentised (I have explained this in No. 41) a process exclusive to homoeopathy.

We use several remedies externally in mother tincture (herbal) form, for instance, **Calendula** for cuts and wounds, **Urtica Urens** for burns.

15. Where do Biochemic remedies fit into Homoeopathy?

They don't.

These remedies are prescribed on the assumption that a disease is caused by a lack of one or more tissue salts. The homoeopathic approach is that there must be an underlying reason for any deficiency and the basic cause should be corrected, thus restoring balance in the economy of the patient.

The fact that these remedies are prepared in accordance with the homoeopathic pharmacopoeia may be responsible for the belief that they are homoeopathic.

Patients having homoeopathic treatment should never take these remedies as they are apt to mask symptoms and thus interfere with the homoeopathic prescription.

It is interesting to note that since the introduction of the 12 original salts by Schussler followers have introduced about two dozen additional substances.

16. Is diet necessary?

Medicine cannot compensate for a bad diet or, indeed, any other bad habit.

There is no so called 'Homoeopathic diet' but Hahnemann, the founder of homoeopathy, said 'Treat the cause' and if incorrect diet is the cause or a contributing factor in ill-health it must be amended.

Dr Dorothy Shepherd stated that vegetarians seemed to respond to homoeopathic remedies better than people who eat meat. I think it wise to advise patients to eat whole foods, plenty of salads, fruit and vegetables, cut sugar consumption to the minimum and avoid all white flour products, junk foods, additives, artificial colouring, flavouring etc. I do not profess to be a dietician but if this is accepted as a way of life it is very beneficial.

17. Do you use remedies in combination?

No, this is the insignia of an incompetent homoeopath.

Combinations of remedies are used extensively on the continent and are now being offered in increasing numbers in this country. They are usually advertised for specific (named) ailments which is contrary to the basic principles of homoeopathy which state that each patient must be treated individually, taking into account both mental and physical symptoms, idiosyncracies etc.

A combination of remedies might include one that will be of help to the patient but so often no improvement is felt and this brings homoeopathy into disrepute.

14

18. Can Homoeopathy alter inherited tendencies?

When treating chronic disease the homoeopath must know as much about 'family history' as possible in order to cure the patient.

So often the indicated remedy does not work as it should and we then have to look into the background for clues. If, for instance, several members of the family have suffered from chest troubles, bronchitis and influenza we then prescribe the medicine which will alter the 'soil' or blood stream which has been inherited, in which these ailments can flourish.

I have described this in simple language because it is difficult to understand but unless the inherited factors are recognised and dealt with many patients can never be cured.

19. Are vitamins necessary?

Theoretically one should obtain all the vitamins necessary from food but these days of processed, convenience foods, often prepared from poor quality ingredients, together with additives etc., it is difficult to live healthily without some supplementary vitamins.

Vitamins are big business and one should avoid being brain-washed into believing that in order to maintain health it is essential to supplement a reasonable diet.

If symptoms indicate a shortage of vitamins then it might be necessary to take a short course of whatever is indicated but even so it is better to try to obtain it through wholesome food. Wholemeal bread, raw salads which include root vegetables such as grated carrot, beetroot etc., and fresh fruit, all organically grown where possible, plus a little protein, should provide most of the elements necessary for health.

There are books giving the vitamin and mineral content of various foods.

20. What is a polychrest?

A remedy covering a wide range of symptoms, it's use is often indicated in the treatment of a deep-seated disease.

21. Can I have Acupuncture at the same time as Homoeopathy?

Both are complete systems of treatment and should never be prescribed at the same time.

I would not be prepared to treat anyone who wished to combine the two because I think that acupuncture might well mask the symptoms on which I would prescribe.

But I would advise anyone who has had unsuccessful treatment by one of the methods to try the other, but not together.

I have seen some results of acupressure and believe that as a first-aid measure it can be most helpful.

22. What is chronic disease?

One that is deep in the economy of the patient and will continue to get worse.

On the other hand an acute condition will clear up in a reasonably short time.

I am sure that you will have heard that a cold is cured in a week if a cold cure is given or in seven days if a little common sense is applied!

23. Do homoeopathic remedies antidote one another?

There are a few remedies that antidote one another and **Camphor** will antidote most homoeopathic medicines but this is an aspect of homoeopathy that is of little importance to the layman because a single remedy should be taken at one time and if it is unsuitable it will either have no effect or its action will cease quickly.

This is an aspect of homoeopathy that has to be taken into consideration by practitioners using high potencies for chronic diseases.

24. How can I study Homoeopathy?

Advice on this aspect is difficult as much depends on how far one wishes to pursue the subject, what time can be devoted to study and whether one is able to absorb knowledge from books.

If the aim is to confine ones efforts to domestic prescribing I suggest *Puddephatt's Primers* and *Homoeopathy, A guide to Natural Medicine* which I wrote to provide a simple outline of the basic principles. These could be followed by a small materia medica such as *Essentials of Homoeopathic Prescribing* by Dr H. Fergie Woods.

In the treatment of children *Homoeopathic Remedies for Children* published recently would be useful as it gives the correct approach to prescribing.

If one wishes to delve more deeply it is necessary to devote a great deal of time to the study of the philosophy of the subject. To begin I recommend *A Study Course in Homoeopathy* which must be studied in conjunction with *The Principles and Art of Cure by Homoeopathy* by Dr H. A. Roberts. Hahnemann's *Organon* (a new translation presented in plain English with the footnotes incorporated in the text has just been published by Gollancz) is a must and Kent's *Lectures on Homoeopathic Philosophy* should also be carefully studied. When the philosophy is understood it is necessary to acquire knowledge of the leading remedies and I suggest Nash's *Leaders in Homoeopathic Therapeutics* and *Homoeopathic Drug Pictures* by Dr Margaret Tyler. I almost forgot to mention Kent's *Lectures* on *Homoeopathic Materia Medica*, a book that should be studied by every homoeopath.

For practical work it is essential to have a repertory and the best is by Kent, it is expensive but the serious prescriber can hardly do without it. At the same time *How to Use the Repertory* by Bidwell teaches how to use this large work correctly.

There are numerous materia medicas for reference and Clarke's *Dictionary of Practical Materia Medica* is the most complete, unfortunately this three volume work is very expensive but there is no substitute.

For those seeking tuition there are a number of schools offering training but it must be borne in mind that the only one officially recognised is confined to qualified doctors, vets and dentists at The Faculty of Homoeopathy.

Anyone considering a training course should make careful enquiries to ensure that the teaching is of a good standard.

25. Is it necessary to study materia medica?

A knowledge of the characteristic symptoms of the leading remedies can be of assistance as it enables a prescription to be made without delay, this is especially useful in injuries and acute troubles.

There are about 2000 remedies in our materia medica although many are seldom used. It may be that under 200 are in daily use, but a study of even this number would involve much time and my advice is to study a dozen or so of the leading medicines; it is better to have a good understanding of a few rather than a superficial knowledge of the action of many. The remedies mentioned in *Puddephatts Primers* are those most likely to be useful.

There are a number of books on first-aid and domestic prescribing which are useful and, with thought, easy to follow.

26. Do you approve of 'The Pill'?

No! The menstrual cycle is a natural function and I believe that anything which interfers with it is harmful.

The ill-effects of such interference may not manifest for a time but I am certain that the long-term effect of taking the pill will be many deep-seated, serious disorders.

When anyone comes to me for help and is taking the pill I do all I can to get them to stop.

27. Do you believe in allergies?

During the last few years allergies seem to have become fashionable!

Extensive tests are undertaken and the patient is told that he is allergic to various foods or substances and advised to abstain from eating them.

Years ago the term was seldom used but occasionally one came across a patient who could not take cheese, eggs or some common food.

The homoeopath believes that when the body is in balance and functioning normally abnormalities such as allergies cannot exist. When a patient asks for help because he has an allergy he is treated as a whole to bring his health to a much higher level when the so-called allergy should disappear.

Here I must add that constitutional treatment should be carried out by an experienced homoeopathic practitioner as many factors have to be taken into consideration and the treatment might be prolonged.

28. Can animals be treated by Homoeopathy?

Homoeopathy is very successful in dealing with all types of animal, many of the more common complaints can be dealt with by those with little or no knowledge of the subject. I have received numerous reports of cures of cats and dogs by the advice given in the simple books on these animals by K. Sheppard.

Naturally, the more serious, deep-seated troubles, should be under the care of a vet. Unfortunately, there are few in the country versed in homoeopathy but the situation is improving and more are studying largely owing to the efforts of George

MacLeod, a veterinary surgeon who has written several excellent books on the treatment of horses, cattle and other animals. Several of my patients have contacted him by letter or telephone and reported that the results have been most satisfactory. Some years ago our cat had worms and a few doses of **Filix Mas.**, in her water soon cleared the trouble. She is over eleven years of age but behaves like a young cat. When off colour **Sulphur** brings her back to normal very quickly. **Sulphur** is probably an excellent remedy for cats as they are philosophical and this remedy is designated as being helpful to 'The ragged philosopher'.

29. Do Homoeopaths approve of vivisection?

No, animals have different mental and physical characteristics according to their species and their reactions are, therefore, likely to differ from those of humans.

All our remedies are tested on healthy human beings and both the mental and physical effects carefully recorded; this is the basis of our materia medica.

The mental state of the patient plays an important part when making a homoeopathic prescription. Experiments on animals do not reveal the finer mental states which are so important to the homoeopath.

Never have animals been used in the 'provings' of homoeopathic remedies.

30. How can I judge the ability of a homoeopathic practitioner?

This is difficult to answer as, in all professions, there are all shades of competence.

In many instances recommendation may be the best guide but, even so, it can be unreliable as all practitioners have success – some more than others.

The only officially recognised degrees in homoeopathy are F.F. Hom., and M.F.Hom., which are confined to doctors, dentists and vets, who have trained in orthodox schools and have subsequently attended The Faculty of Homoeopathy.

Many homoeopathic doctors practice under the NHS, but they are usually very busy and unable to devote more than a few minutes to each patient. In injuries and acute troubles this may be sufficient but the more deep-seated, chronic diseases usually require a consultation lasting about an hour.

Others have a full-time homoeopathic practise usually giving an hour for the first consultation. There are, also, some extremely good lay homoeopaths.

As one acquires knowledge of homoeopathy the more one is able to judge the ability of the prescriber by his questions and the manner in which they are put.

I'm sorry there is no simple answer to this question.

31. What is the usual dosage in Homoeopathy?

There is not set dosage but one pill or tablet is all that is necessary, more would have no greater effect.

Homoeopathic remedies do not rely upon quantity as their preparation by potentisation releases the inherent powers from the crude substance which, for want of a better description, might be called 'energy'. No form of analysis can detect any material substance in potencies above the 9th or 10th yet the high potencies can have dramatic effects.

The repetition of the dose depends entirely upon the case, in some injuries it might be necessary to give the remedy every few minutes until a reaction is obtained. In many ailments 3 times a day is sufficient and in constitutional prescribing one dose of a high potency may work for a month or longer.

Always bear in mind that a remedy should never be repeated as long as improvement is taking place, repeat only when the patient slips back and old symptoms return. If new ones develop then another remedy must be found to match them.

32. Where should I purchase homoeopathic remedies and in what form?

The preparation and storage of remedies is of great importance and you should always obtain the products of a firm specialising in homoeopathic pharmacy even if they are a little more expensive than those of other firms. A well experienced firm prepare remedies from the correct basic source. Dr Tyler in her excellent *Homoeopathic Drug Pictures* devotes space to the importance of obtaining remedies from a reliable source. A limited range of remedies is now stocked by some chemists and health food stores and as long as they are kept away from strong perfumes in a cool place they should be satisfactory. I have had no experience of these remedies as I always obtain supplies from Ainsworth's Homoeopathic Pharmacy in London, a firm that holds the Royal Warrant. They give a very efficient postal service and I am informed that The Galen Pharmacy of Dorchester supplies west country customers promptly.

Most chemists supply remedies in tablet form and this seems to be satisfactory but some firms will prepare in pill or liquid form if specially asked to do so. The form is unimportant, one pill, tablet or drop is a dose.

Where it is impossible to administer the remedy in pill or tablet form, as in the case of a newly born baby, dissolve one pill or two, or a crushed tablet in a little cold water, stir and give a sip from a spoon.

33. Which is the best way to store homoeopathic remedies?

As homoeopathic remedies are susceptible to outside influences they should be kept in a reasonably cool place away from strong sunlight, preferably in a drawer, and especial care should be taken to ensure that they are well away from all strong smelling substances such as perfumes, camphor, peppermint, strongly scented soap, lipstick etc. Never transfer a remedy from one bottle to another that has contained a different remedy or potency.

34. How long do homoeopathic remedies last?

There is no time limit when properly stored.

Although I have heard suggestions that they should be renewed every ten years I am still using remedies that are at least 50 years old and they still work as efficiently as ever.

35. Can you advise on the most suitable books?

The answer to this depends upon the extent to which you wish to use homoeopathy and the time you can devote to study.

As I have already answered a question in regard to the study of the subject I will mention a few simple works.

As **Arnica** is the most widely used remedy which should be carried about by everyone, the beginner should know the wide range of troubles it can help. I wrote a little book about this remedy many years ago called *Arnica the Wonder Herb* because I felt that it was so important. This book is still available. *Before Calling the Doctor* gives the main remedies for common ailments and it is simple to use.

The British Homoeopathic Association issues Dr D. M. Gibson's *First Aid Homoeopathy in Accidents & Ailments* which is very good and *Homoeopathic Medicine at Home* by Dr Panos & Heimlich, an American publication issued in this country by Corgi is somewhat larger but very helpful.

Dr Dorothy Shepherd's *Homoeopathy for the First Aider* is another practical book giving details for the use of the more common remedies in an interesting manner.

Lastly, I am working on a new book dealing with emergencies which will be published by Health Science Press under the title

Homeopathy for Emergencies. It should be helpful to beginners and those with little knowledge of the subject as it indicates both potency and dosage for injuries and common ailments.

36. How can I become a practitioner?

My answer to *How can I study homoeopathy?* does, I think, answer this question.

There is nothing to prevent anyone in this country setting up as a homoeopathic practitioner irrespective of their knowledge of the subject. This, I believe, puts an enormous onus on the would-be practitioner – he should love people, love homoeopathy and remember that he is dealing with the most important part of creation – human beings. Homoeopathy is a vast subject and one never stops learning.

A great deal of 'toil, sweat and tears' goes into the training but if one stays the course I can say, after 30 years experience 'It has all been so worthwhile'.

37. How long should a homoeopathic consultation last?

On average the first consultation lasts about an hour when dealing with a chronic ailment. Where there is an injury or an acute condition a few minutes will usually suffice.

A chronic case has to be thoroughly investigated, and the patients full medical history recorded. We need to find out about his or her reaction to weather, food and drink; if they have had many vaccinations and inoculations and most important of all whether through the illness they have become very depressed, sensitive, angry, jealous and so on.

Having the details on a case-paper enables the practitioner to check the effects of the prescription and any alteration in the condition of the patient to the second and subsequent consultations might last up to half-an-hour.

I would mention that having taken the case in detail it is then necessary for the prescriber to analyse the details and then repertorize the relavent symptoms before making a prescription. Depending on the case this can take much time, sometimes more than an hour.

38. Is homoeopathy practised by NHS doctors?

Yes, there is an increasing number of fully qualified doctors prescribing homoeopathic medicines and addresses can be supplied by The British Homoeopathic Association and other bodies.

These doctors are undoubtedly successful in many acute ailments and injuries but there can be difficulty in dealing with chronic troubles which require prolonged investigation as, under the NHS they are usually very busy caring for a great number of patients and it is impossible to devote sufficient time to take the case fully.

There are doctors who can be consultated privately but they are mainly in London.

39. What is your attitude towards Radionics?

I am dedicated to the Hahnemannian approach to treatment and believe that the most satisfactory way in which to find the similimum is by the laborious repertorization of symptoms.

Practitioners of radiesthesia and radionics often claim to have discovered latent troubles and, subsequently, to have eliminated them although there can be no scientific confirmation that they ever existed.

At times these methods seem to achieve spectacular results but I would always prefer to rely upon the purely homoeopathic approach.

40. Which half-a-dozen remedies would you advise to start a small medicine chest?

Arnica 30 must be the first as it deal with bruises of the muscles and should always be given in an accident as it removes the shock from the physical injury. Every simple book on homoeopathy gives details for the use of this and other remedies that can be used for common troubles.

Other remedies could be **Calendula** Ø (the sign indicates mother tincture) for external application to cuts, it is the finest healing agent. **Aconite 12** is often needed by children whose ailments come on suddenly after being exposed to cold winds; they are fearful and restless.

Nux Vomica has many uses (as have all our remedies); the patient is very irritable, feels terrible in the morning after too much food and drink; feels cold and develops symptoms, he cannot get warm even with added clothing and by a fire.

Arsenicum for chills with restlessness so that he cannot stay in one place for long, must be kept warm except his head which needs cool air. Also for tummy upsets, when symptoms agree and ptomaine poisoning.

Pulsatilla for **ANY** symptoms which are better walking around slowly in fresh air – must have air – patient cannot eat any fatty foods, often weepy and loves consolation.

The last 3 remedies are recommended in the 12th potency.

41. What exactly is potentisation?

Hahnemann found the administration of crude substances unsatisfactory and he sought a scientific way of dilution.

To one drop of the original substance (mother tincture) he added 99 drops of diluent (usually distilled water) and shook it vigorously; this made the first potency (1 or 1c following the name of the remedy). He then took one drop of the first (1c) potency, added 99 drops of diluent and after shaking as before obtained the second (2 or 2c) potency. Each potency was prepared in the same manner, one drop of the previous potency to 99 drops of diluent.

Hahnemann prepared remedies up to the 30th diluation but since his time the 200th, 1m, 10m and even higher have been made and used with excellent results.

It is difficult to describe potentisation in simple language but, briefly, more and more energy of the substance is released by each step and, therefore, the remedy becomes more powerful.

Obviously, the 200th and higher potencies must always be used with care and discretion and they should at all times be prescribed by experienced homoeopaths.

Remedies are also prepared on the decimal scale (1 in 10) and so we have 3x, 6x, 12x and so on. These are not as popular as the centesimal potencies in this country.

42. Do you approve of vaccination and immunization?

This is a very thorny question as some homoeopathic physicians are in favour of both.

I disapprove of the injection of any foreign substance into a healthy body as I believe that anyone in good health can resist epidemics. Homoeopathy when correctly prescribed raises the persons health. A very famous homoeopath, Dr J. Compton Burnett, wrote a book call *Vaccinosis* in which he gave details of many ailments caused by vaccination which baffled those who were ignorant of the dangers of this practice.

Although there are occasional reports of serious troubles or death caused by allopathic immunizations we hear nothing of the 'mystery' symptoms which occur in many cases long afterwards. Fortunately homoeopathy can deal with and eliminate the injurious results.

I always question every patient closely about vaccinations and immunizations and if I suspect they might be a factor in the disease I prescribe with this in mind.

Various books mention the risks involved in these practices, one is *Health Shock* by Martin Weitz which has been issued in paperback. It also includes details of the ill-effects of numerous drugs, many of which are readily available in chemists.

The individual must make up his own mind as to whether the risk is worthwhile. My husband has compiled a small book called *Homoeopathy and Immunization* giving the homoeopathic alternatives which is a help to those who need more information.